Rose Infused Radiance

A guide to DIY Skincare with Roses

by Carrie Scharf

Index

Disclaimer: The information in this book is not intended to treat, cure, diagnose, or otherwise address medical conditions or ailments. This book is for educational, entertainment, and informational purposes only.

The contents of this book have been thoroughly reviewed for accuracy. However, the author disclaims any liability for any damages, losses, or injuries that may result from the use or misuse of any product or information presented herein. It is the purchaser's responsibility to read and follow all instructions and warnings on all product labels.

Roses

A few days ago someone told me that they didn't realize it was so simple to make rose water. What I hope that you get from this book is that all-natural skincare can be simple and inexpensive and can leave you with healthy, beautiful skin. I also want you to be able to transform your bath time into a cozy retreat with luxurious rose milk baths, leaving your skin feeling soft and nourished. I want you to treat yourself to a pampering rose body scrub, gently exfoliating away dull skin to reveal a radiant complexion.

Why use roses? Roses are antibacterial and anti-inflammatory. They are high in tannins and gallic acid (antioxidant) and linoleic acid (omega 6). They also have Alpha-linolenic acid (omega 3), pro-vitamin A and vitamins C and E.

Roses are moisturizing, relaxing, and toning. They are great for sensitive, weak and mature skin. They are a good wrinkle eraser, redness soother, and oil reducer. They help protect against free radicals and assist in the production of collagen. Roses help skin's brightness and tone, help pores appear smaller, and even diminish acne scars.

Gather the buds when they are formed. Gather the petals when they are first opened. Gather the rose hips when they are ripe.

I'd love to hear about your creations. You can find me at www.skincarecookbook.com or www.carrieshandmadeessentials.com. There, you can take my free e-course, read my articles, or learn about my memberships.

Rose Water For Skin and Hair

To make rose water at home, you'll need rose petals (fresh or dried), distilled water, and a pot with a lid. To use rose water, you can use it on your skin as a toner, use it in skincare recipes, or add it to your bathwater for a relaxing experience.

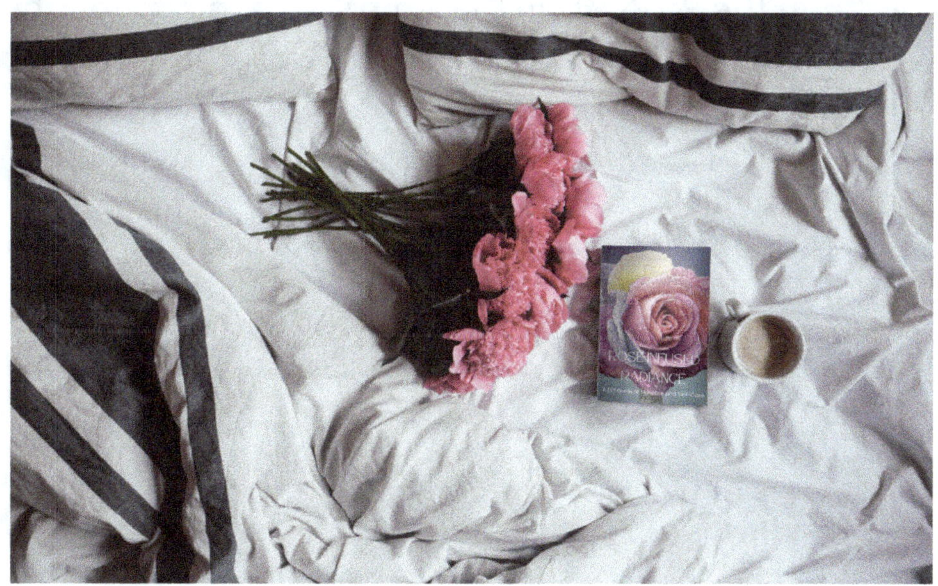

How to Make Rose Water for Skin and Hair

Directions:

Pick Rose Petals: Pick about 2 cups of fresh rose petals. Make sure they are clean and have not been sprayed with pesticides.

Rinse the Petals: Gently rinse your roses with cold water to remove any dirt or bugs.

Boil Water: In a pot, bring 2 cups of distilled water to a simmer. Do not bring it to a rolling boil.

Add In Your Rose Petals: Put your rose petals in the simmering water. Put a lid on the pot and let it simmer for about 20-30 minutes, or until the petals have lost their color.

Strain the Roses from the Water: Take the pot off the heat and let it cool a little while. Strain the liquid into a clean glass jar or bottle.

Storing Rose Water: Store rose water in the refrigerator for up to a week. You can also add a few drops of rose essential oil to make the rose fragrance stronger.

The Benefits of Rose Water for Skin and Hair

For Skin:

Hydration

Rose water is great for dry or dehydrated skin as it is very hydrating and moisturizing.

Roses are Toning

Roses have astringent and anti-inflammatory properties and are a great ingredient to help tone and tighten the pores.

Roses Help Bring Balance

Rose water helps balance the pH of the skin which makes it useful for all skin types.

Roses are Soothing

Roses have anti-inflammatory properties that can help calm irritation and redness.

Roses are Antioxidant

Rose water contains antioxidants that help protect the skin from damage caused by free radicals.

Roses are Anti-aging

Roses can help reduce the appearance of fine lines and wrinkles, giving the skin a more youthful appearance.

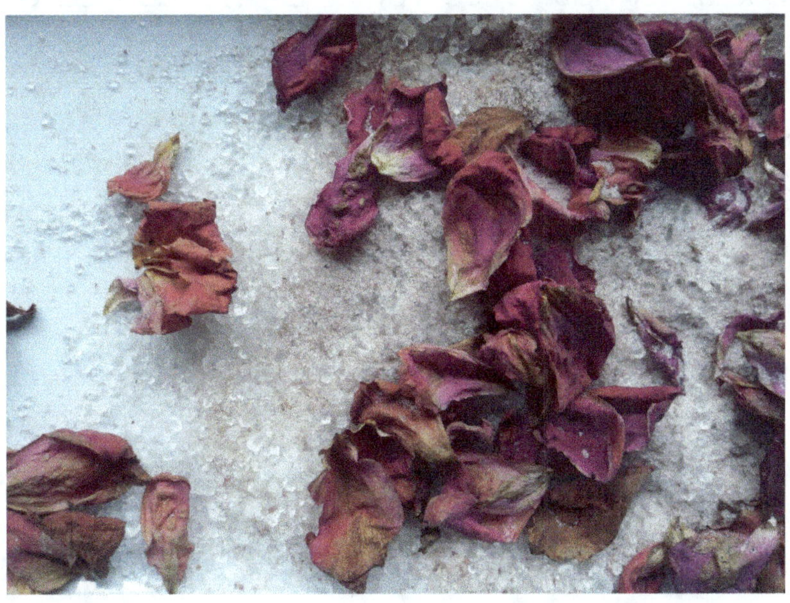

For Hair:

Roses are Conditioning

Rose water can help condition the hair, which makes it softer and more manageable.

Roses are Good for Scalp Health

Roses contain vitamins A, B3, C, and E can help with an irritated scalp and promote healthy hair growth.

Roses Make Hair Shine

Rose water moisturizes and hydrates which can add a shine to the hair, making it look smoother, healthier and more vibrant.

Roses Smell Lovely

Rose water has a nice fragrance that can leave your hair smelling great.

Roses are Refreshing

Spraying rose water on your hair can refresh and revive it, especially on hot days or after a workout. It is great to use on your body as well.

10 Ways to Use Rose Water

Rose water is a versatile ingredient that can benefit both the skin and hair. Here are 10 ways to use rose water:

Facial Toner

After cleansing, apply rose water to your face in a spray bottle or using a cotton pad to tone and hydrate the skin.

Makeup Setting Spray

Use rose water as a natural setting spray to help set your makeup. Make your own by using 1 teaspoon of rose water, 1 teaspoon of witch hazel, and 1 ½ cups water. Keep it for 2-3 weeks in the refrigerator.

Hydrating Mist

Spray rose water on your face throughout the day to refresh and cool your skin.

Hair Rinse

After shampooing, rinse your hair with rose water to condition and add shine.

Scalp Treatment

Massage rose water into your scalp to soothe irritation and promote healthy hair growth.

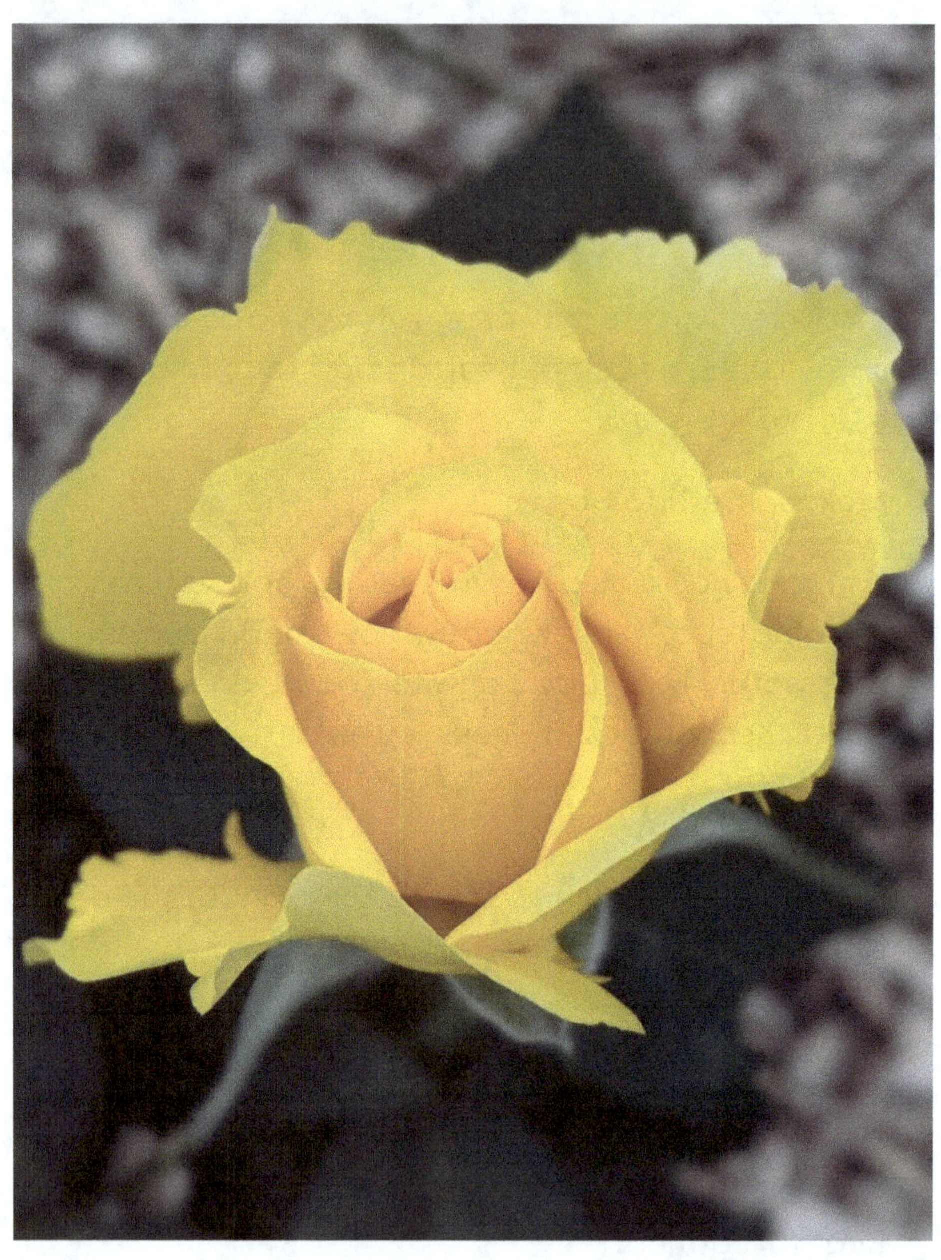

For the Bath

Add rose water to your bathwater for a relaxing and aromatic bathtime. Some essential oils that go well with rose are: bergamot, chamomile, clary sage, fennel, geranium, lavender, lemon, neroli, patchouli, sandalwood, and ylang-ylang.

Face Mask

Mix rose water with clay or other ingredients to create a hydrating and soothing face mask. See recipe below.

Sunburn Relief

Spray rose water on sunburned skin to soothe irritation and reduce redness. See recipe below.

Eye Compress

Soak cotton pads in rose water and place them over your eyes to reduce puffiness and refresh tired eyes.

Aromatherapy

Inhaling the scent of rose water can help you relax and reduce stress.

Soothing Sunburn Spray

To make a soothing sunburn spray with rose water, you'll need a few simple ingredients.

Ingredients:

1/2 cup rose water

2 tablespoons aloe vera gel

1 tablespoon witch hazel

5-10 drops lavender essential oil (optional, for extra healing power)

You could also try these essential oil blends: lavender and peppermint, lavender and roman chamomile, frankincense and helichrysum, and lavender and tea tree.

Directions:

1. In a spray bottle, combine the rose water, aloe vera gel, witch hazel, and essential oils.
2. Shake the bottle well to mix all the ingredients thoroughly.
3. To use, shake the bottle and spray the sunburn spray onto the affected area of your skin. Avoid spraying it in your eyes.
4. Allow the spray to air dry and reapply as needed for relief.

Face Mask

Ingredients:

2 tablespoons rose water

1 tablespoon honey

1 tablespoon yogurt (plain, unsweetened)

Directions:

1. In a small bowl, mix together the rose water, honey, and yogurt until well combined.
2. Apply the mixture to your clean face, avoiding the eye area.
3. Leave the mask on for about 15-20 minutes.
4. Rinse off with lukewarm water and pat your skin dry.
5. Follow up with your favorite moisturizer.

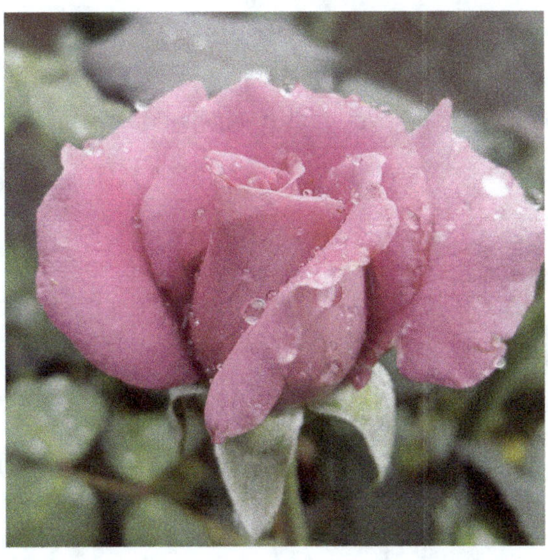

Hydrosols or Decoctions?

Which should you use?

The answer depends on the needs of your skin and what you want to use it for.

For skincare purposes, hydrosols are mild, and they can hydrate and tone the skin.

Decoctions are stronger and more potent than hydrosols, but they do not contain essential oils like hydrosols do.

What is a hydrosol?

Hydrosols or hydrolats or floral waters are made through steam distillation. They mostly contain hydrophilic compounds of the plant with a tiny amount of essential oil compounds.

Hydrosols are a great way to get the benefits of an expensive essential oil but without spending the money. For instance, rose essential oil is expensive but you can take a few roses out of your garden and make a rose hydrosol.

You can use a hydrosol anywhere undiluted as they are very gentle. They are loved because they are hydrating, soothing and refreshing.

How to Make a Hydrosol

Directions:

1. In a large pot, put one heat safe bowl upside down with a smaller heat safe bowl right side up on top of it.
2. Place about 5 cups of dried or fresh plant material around the bowl.
3. Cover plant material with water. Do not let water level go above the top of the bigger bowl.
4. Put the pot lid on upside down. Put a freezer bag filled with ice on top of the lid.
5. Boil the water and simmer for at least 30 minutes. Replace the ice in the bag when it melts.
6. Take the pot off the burner and remove the lid. The small bowl will contain the hydrosol. Pour the water in a dark bottle or jar. Store in a cool, dark place.

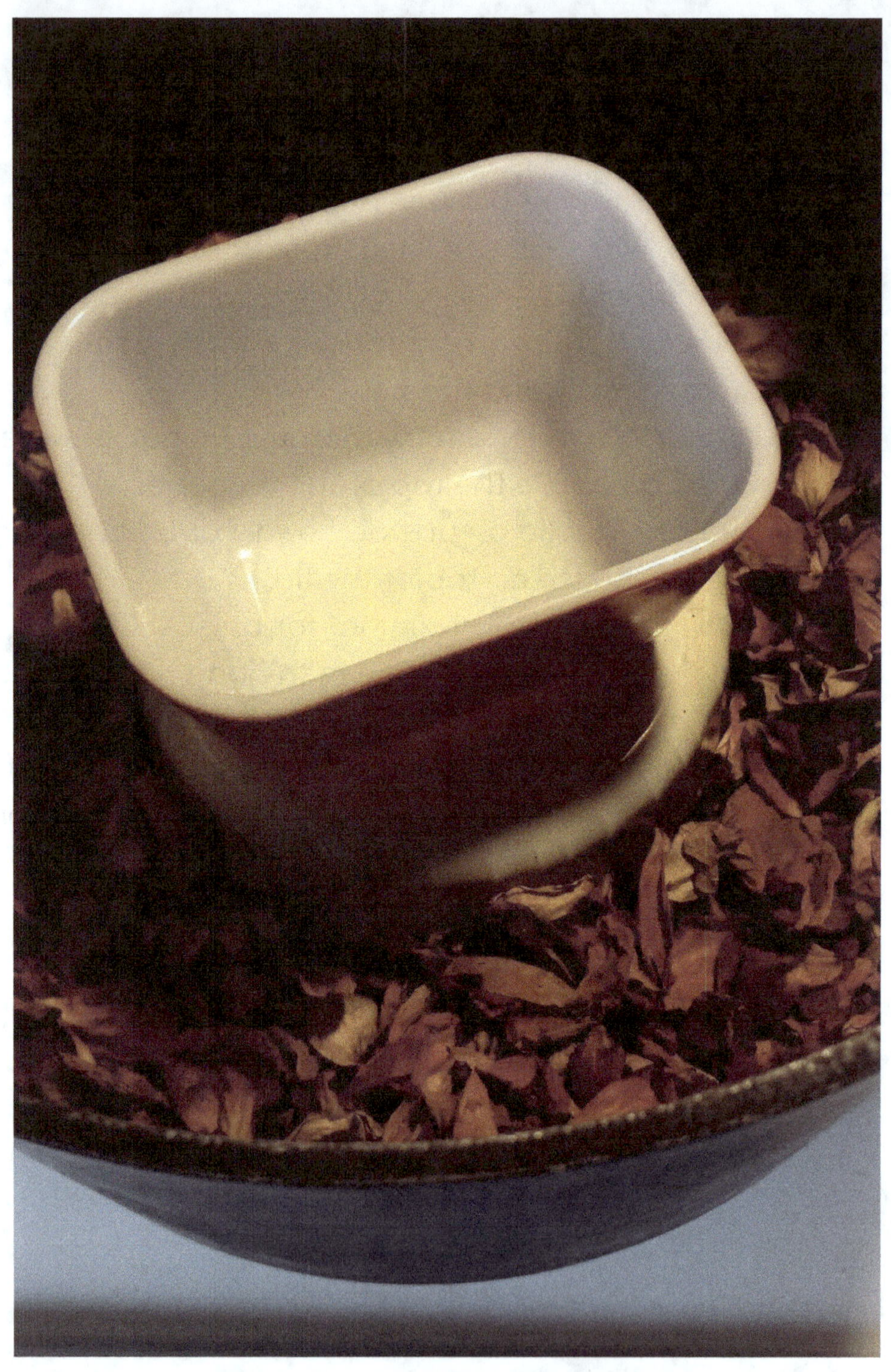

Ways to Use a Hydrosol

Hydrosols, also known as floral waters, can be a versatile addition to your self-care routine. If you have sensitive skin, you might want to do a patch test to make sure you are not allergic or sensitive to the botanicals you are using.

Some ways I like to use hydrosols are:

Toner

Hydrosols make excellent natural facial toners. You can use them by themselves or add things like glycerin, witch hazel, aloe, and essential oils. Spray this refreshing spray onto clean skin after your cleanser or apply with a cotton pad to help hydrate, refresh, and balance the skin's ph.

Body Mist

Use hydrosols as a refreshing body mist. Spray your skin after a shower or anytime you need a pick-me-up.

Hair Refresher

Spray hydrosols onto your hair to refresh and add a subtle fragrance. They can also help condition and add shine to your hair. See the recipe below.

Aromatherapy

Use hydrosols as aromatherapy. Spray them anywhere like your car or linens or on a tissue for a gentle, natural scent that can uplift your mood or help you relax. Add essential oils if you wish.

Compress

Soak a cloth in chilled hydrosol and apply it as a compress to tired eyes, a sunburn, or a headache for a soothing effect.

In the Bathtub

Add some hydrosol to your bathwater for a relaxing bath with a lovely scent.

Room Spray

Use hydrosols as a natural room spray to freshen up your living space.

Natural Perfume

Use hydrosols as a natural, subtle perfume by spraying them lightly on your skin.

Ingredient in Your Skincare Recipes

Use hydrosols as an ingredient in your skincare creations such as bath tea, lotions, and masks for their beneficial properties.

Hydrating Mist

Keep a spray bottle of hydrosol in your bag and use it as a hydrating mist throughout the day, especially in places that are hot and dry. You can add some peppermint and eucalyptus and make it a cooling spray.

Decoctions

Decoctions are made by boiling plant material, such as roots, bark, petals, leaves, or seeds, in water to extract their active compounds. Decoctions are more concentrated than hydrosols and are often used for their medicinal properties. You can drink it as a tea or use it on your skin. They are usually stronger than a tea which we would call an infusion as they are cooked for a longer time to make sure we extract all their wonderful properties.

How to Make a Decoction

To make a decoction, follow these steps:

1. **Choose Your botanicals:** Select the herbs, roots, barks, or seeds you want to use for your decoction.
2. **Prepare Your Ingredients:** If using roots, barks, or seeds, chop or crush them to increase the surface area. If using dried herbs, crush them slightly to release their oils.

3. **Measure:** Use about 1 tablespoon of dried herbs or 2 tablespoons of fresh herbs per cup of water.
4. **Boil the Water:** In a saucepan, bring the water to a boil.
5. **Add the botanicals:** Add the herbs or flowers to the boiling water.
6. **Simmer:** Reduce the heat to low and let the herbs simmer in the water for about 15-30 minutes depending on how strong you want it.
7. **Strain:** Take the pan off of the heat and strain the liquid into a bowl using a fine-mesh strainer or cheesecloth.
8. **Cool:** Let your decoction cool.
9. **Store:** Store any unused decoction in the refrigerator for up to a few days. You can also freeze it in ice cube trays.

Ways to Use a Decoction

Decoctions are useful in many ways. Make sure that the plant matter you are using is safe for the reason you want to use it and that you are not allergic to it. Also, do not use plants that have been sprayed with pesticides. So, you probably don't want to use the roses that you were given for your birthday. Here are some ways you can use a decoction:

Facial Steam

Add your decoction to a bowl of hot water and use it for a facial steam. This can help open up pores, cleanse the skin, and promote relaxation.

Hair Rinse

Use your decoction as a final rinse after washing your hair. It can help condition the hair, promote shine, and soothe the scalp. See the recipe below.

Foot Soak

Add your decoction to a basin of warm water and soak your feet. This can help relieve tired, achy feet and soften the skin.

Compress

Soak a cloth in your decoction and apply it as a warm or cold compress to areas of the body that need relief, such as sore muscles or joints.

Mouth Rinse

Use your decoction as a mouth rinse to help freshen breath, soothe gum inflammation, or relieve toothache.

Add to Your Bath

Add your decoction to your bathwater for a relaxing soak. This can help nourish the skin and promote overall relaxation.

Inhalation

Add your decoction to a bowl of hot water and inhale the steam to help relieve congestion or sinus pressure. Add essential oils such as peppermint, lavender or eucalyptus.

Face and Body Spray

Using a funnel, pour your decoction to a spray bottle and use it as a refreshing spray for the face or body.

Skincare Products

Use your decoction in homemade skincare products such as lotions, creams, or balms for added nourishment and benefits.

Rose Chamomile Hair Rinse

This hair rinse can help to condition and soften your hair. Adjust the strength of the infusion by using more or less flowers, depending on your hair's needs and your personal preference.

Ingredients:

- 2 tablespoons dried rose petals
- 2 tablespoons dried chamomile flowers
- 2 cups water

Directions:

1. In a small pan, bring the water to a boil.
2. Take the pan off the heat and add the dried rose petals and chamomile flowers.
3. Cover the pan and let the herbs steep for about 30 minutes.
4. Strain the mixture to remove the herbs and pour the infused water into a glass jar.
5. To use, shampoo your hair as usual, then pour the rose chamomile hair rinse over your hair, making sure to saturate it completely.
6. Leave the rinse in your hair for a few minutes, then rinse it out thoroughly with water.

Rose Hair Refresher

To make a floral hair refresher that will hydrate and revitalize your hair, you'll need a rose hydrosol and essential oils (optional).

Ingredients:

- 1/2 cup rose hydrosol
- 1/4 cup distilled water
- 5-10 drops of essential oils (optional, for fragrance)

Here are some essential oil blends you might like to try: 1) chamomile, lavender, and sandalwood, 2) Rosemary, tea tree, eucalyptus, 3) geranium, ylang-ylang, and jasmine, 4) orange, lemon, bergamot, and 5) lavender, rosemary, and peppermint.

Directions:

1. In a clean spray bottle, combine the rose hydrosol and distilled water.
2. Add a few drops of essential oils if you think the hydrosol fragrance is not strong enough.
3. Shake the bottle well to mix the ingredients.
4. To use, shake the bottle and spray onto dry hair, focusing on the roots and lengths.
5. Allow the hair refresher to air dry, or gently pat your hair to help it absorb the spray.

Making a Rose Infused Oil

How to make an oil infusion

There are a few different ways to infuse oils. You can infuse them with the sun, the stove, a slow cooker or the oven. I usually use a slow cooker as I want to do it fairly quickly. Start with a sterilized jar with an airtight lid. Fill it ½ to ¾ of the way with dried flowers. Pour in oil to cover the flowers. Mix so that no air bubbles remain. Cover with a piece of wax paper (to protect from chemicals on the lid) and place the lid on.

Cold Infusion Method

To use the cold infused method, put the container in a sunny windowsill for 4 to 6 weeks, shaking the bottle every few days.

To Infuse in the Slow Cooker

To infuse in the slow cooker, place the sealed jar in a slow cooker and cook for 4 to 8 hours. Be sure to keep an eye on the water level to keep water covering the jar.

To Infuse on the Stove

To use the stove, put herbs and oil without a lid in a double boiler and cook for 30 to 60 minutes. Be careful so that you do not splash water into the oil mixture. Be sure to watch the water level.

To Infuse in the Oven

For the oven infusion, preheat the oven to 120-140 degrees Fahrenheit. Put mixture into a sterilized oven safe dish and bake uncovered for 4 to 8 hours.

When the Process is Done

When the infusing process is done, strain the oil into a clean sterilized jar and store in a cool, dark place of your choice. Pour in oil to cover the flowers or leaves. Mix so that there are no air bubbles.

Why use Body Oil?

I use body oil every day instead of lotion. This is because oil is more easily absorbed into the skin as the body recognizes it and knows what to do with it. Thus, keeping moisture in and nourishing your skin.

Using vegetable or nut-based oils, such as jojoba, almond, and avocado oils, are the best way to ensure that you are truly feeding your skin important nutrients. Dermatologists recommend oils for acne ridden and oily skin because these oils help to regulate sebum production. (Sebum is the oil your body creates to protect and moisturize your skin.) Plus, oils tend to be cleaner, having less fillers and toxic ingredients.

There are so many wonderful plants you can infuse your body oils with. Use plants to soothe skin with plants like lavender or chamomile. You can make oils or balms to help itchy skin or help heal boo-boos. You can use your infused oils directly in the bath or mix them with salts or bath tea.

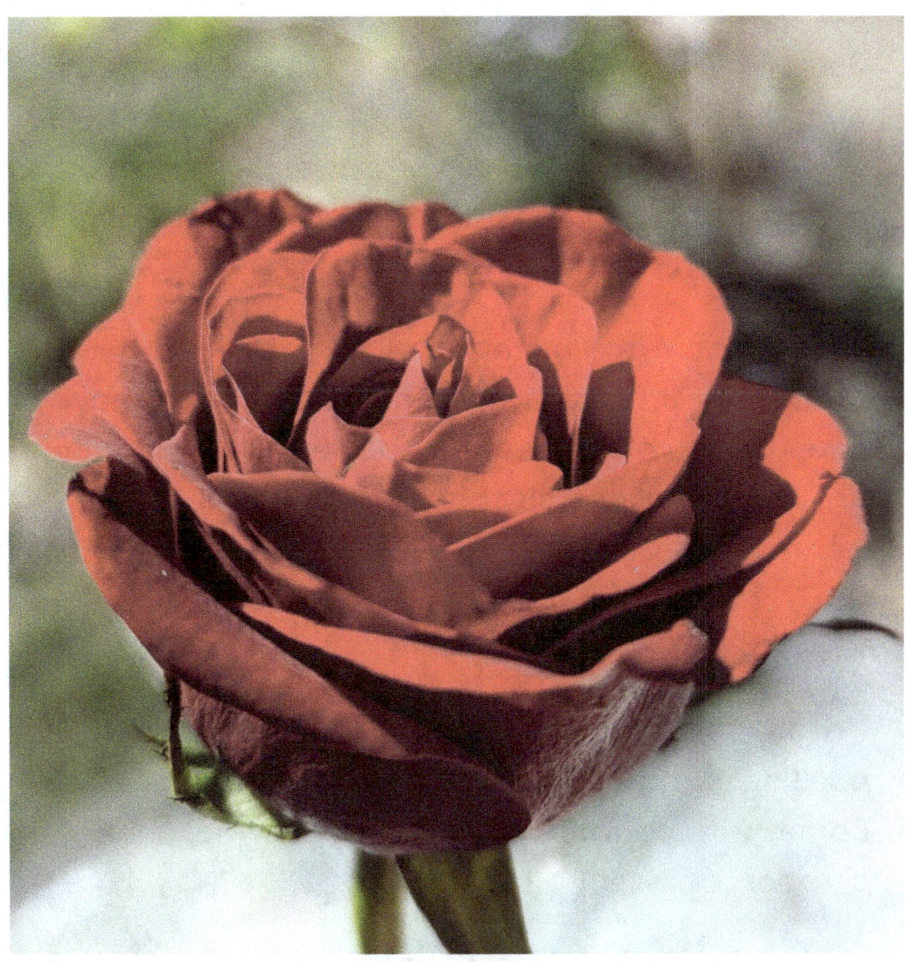

Making a Rose Witch Hazel Infusion

To make a rose witch hazel infusion, dry rose petals and put them in a glass jar. Fill the jar with witch hazel and let it sit for a week before straining.

What is Witch Hazel and Why Should I Use it?

Witch hazel, derived from the leaves and bark of the witch hazel plant (Hamamelis virginiana), has been used for centuries for its various skincare benefits. Here are some of the potential advantages of using witch hazel for the skin:

Astringent: Witch hazel is well-known for its astringent properties. It helps tighten and tone the skin by constricting blood vessels and reducing inflammation. This can be especially beneficial for individuals with oily or acne-prone skin.

Anti-Inflammatory: The natural anti-inflammatory properties of witch hazel make it effective in soothing irritated skin. It may help get rid of redness and swelling. It may also help with the discomfort that comes with conditions like acne, eczema, cuts and scrapes, or insect bites.

Antioxidant: Witch hazel contains tannins which have antioxidant properties that help neutralize free radicals. Free radicals contribute to premature aging and skin damage,

Gentle Cleansing: Witch hazel can be used as a gentle cleanser. Use it to remove excess oil, dirt, and impurities from the skin. It is more mild than traditional alcohol-based toners, which makes it good to use on various skin types, including sensitive skin.

Reducing Puffiness: The astringent properties of witch hazel make it helpful in reducing puffiness and swelling. Use it for under-eye bags or tired-looking eyes.

Soothing Sunburn: Witch hazel is a good choice for soothing sunburn because of its anti-inflammatory and cooling properties. Ease discomfort and help redness by applying witch hazel to sun-exposed skin.

Hydration without Oiliness: Witch hazel can hydrate skin without leaving an oily residue. Therefore it can be used on combination or oily skin for those who want to maintain moisture balance.

Supporting Wound Healing: Apply witch hazel to cuts, bruises, or abrasions as its astringent and anti-inflammatory properties may aid in the healing process. It can help cleanse the wound and reduce inflammation.

Calming Razor Burn: Apply witch hazel to the skin after shaving to help soothe razor burn irritation. Because of these soothing properties, it is often an ingredient in aftershave products.

Rose Cleansing Water

To make a cleansing water using rose-infused witch hazel, you'll need a few simple ingredients. Here's a basic recipe:

Ingredients:

- 1/4 cup rose-infused witch hazel
- 3/4 cup distilled water
- 1 teaspoon vegetable glycerin
- 1-2 drops gentle liquid soap (optional, for cleansing)

Directions:

1. Mix the rose-infused witch hazel, distilled water, and vegetable glycerin in a clean container. Stir well to combine.
2. If you'd like to add a cleansing element, stir in 1-2 drops of gentle liquid soap. Be careful not to add too much, as it can be drying to the skin.
3. Pour your mixture into a clean bottle with a spray or pour cap for easy use.
4. To use, shake the bottle well, then apply the cleansing water to a cotton pad and gently swipe it over your face to cleanse and refresh your skin.
5. Then apply your favorite moisturizer.

This cleansing water can be customized based on your skin's needs. You can change the amount of witch hazel, add different essential oils for their skin benefits, or leave out the glycerin or soap if you would like a simpler formula.

Rose Facial Mist:

Directions:

- 1/2 cup rose-infused witch hazel
- 1/4 cup distilled water
- 1 tablespoon aloe vera gel
- 5-10 drops rose otto or rose geranium essential oil

Directions

1. In a clean spray bottle, combine the rose-infused witch hazel, distilled water, and aloe vera gel.
2. Add the essential oil, if using, and shake the bottle well to mix all the ingredients.
3. Store the bottle in a cool, dark place.
4. To use, shake the bottle well, then spray the mist onto your face with your eyes closed. Allow it to air dry or gently pat it into your skin.
5. You can use this mist throughout the day to hydrate and refresh your skin, or as a setting spray after applying makeup.

Feel free to adjust the ratio of witch hazel to water or add more or less aloe vera gel based on your skin's needs.

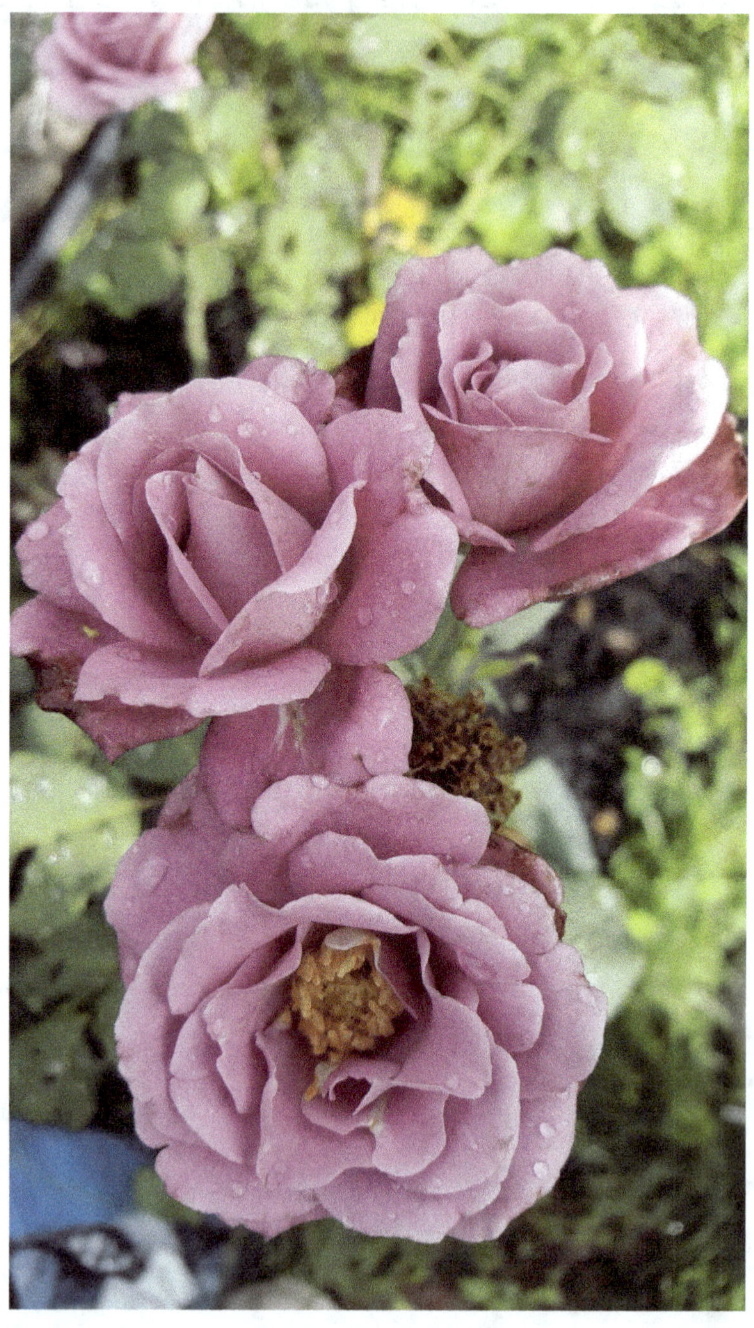

Making a Rose Infused Vinegar

Start by using a clean and sterilized jar. Fill it with roses or whatever other plant or herb you would like. The more herbs, the stronger the infusion. Pour enough apple cider vinegar to cover the flower petals.

Pack the rose petals down with a wooden spoon. Crushing the rose petals will help the infusion. If there's extra room in the jar, add more rose petals. Close the jar with a plastic lid (vinegar will corrode the metal) and store in a cool, dry place for at least 2 weeks. Gently shake the mixture every couple of days. Let it sit longer for a stronger, darker infusion. Strain the roses from the liquid and keep it in a dark glass container.

Uses

Try using your rose infused vinegar for:

A Hair Rinse: Dilute rose-infused vinegar with water (about 1 part vinegar to 2 parts water) and use it as a final rinse after shampooing to help condition and add shine to your hair.

A Facial Toner: Mix rose-infused vinegar with distilled water (about 1 part vinegar to 3 parts water) and use it as a facial toner to help balance the skin's pH and tighten pores.

For Sunburn Relief: Dilute rose-infused vinegar with water and spray or dab it onto sunburned skin to help soothe and relieve discomfort.

A Foot Soak: Add a few tablespoons of rose-infused vinegar to a foot soak to help refresh tired feet and reduce odor.

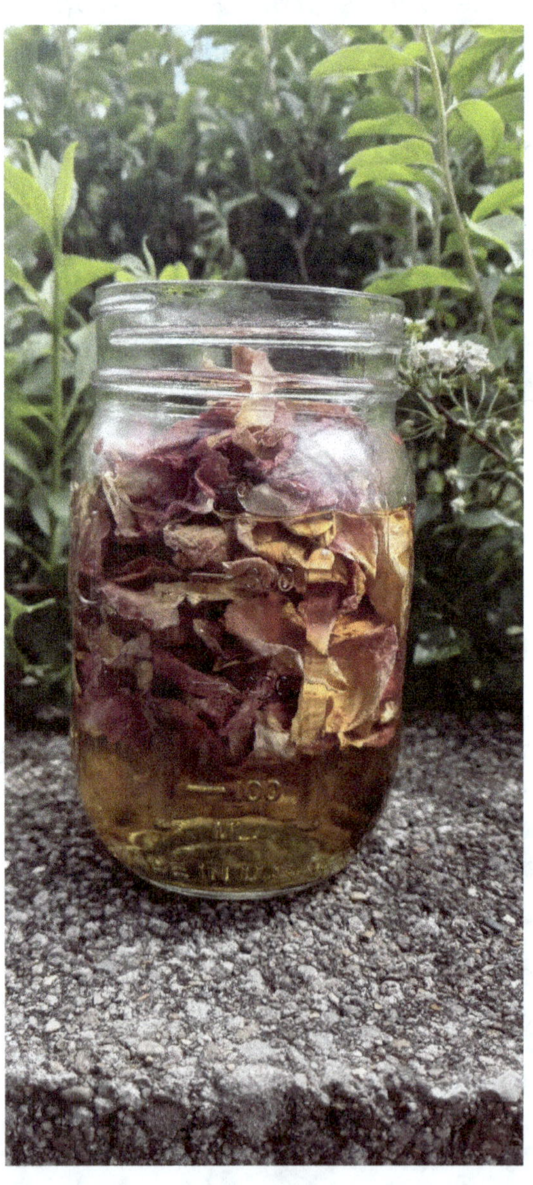

Cleanse and Hydrate your Face Naturally

Rose Honey Facial Cleanser

Ingredients:

- 1/3 cup honey.
- 1/3 cup liquid castile soap.
- 3 tablespoons rose water.
- 2 tablespoons of your favorite oil.

Directions:

In a soap dispenser, first add the rose water, then the liquid castile soap, honey, and oil. Put the top on and shake until the honey is fully dissolved.

You may use your cleanser right away, or store in a cool place to use later. Store the honey soap for up to a month. It's important to use distilled water because tap water will quickly grow mold and bacteria within a few days.

Aloe Toner

- 1/2 cup rose water.
- 1/2 cup aloe vera.

Mix together thorouhgly, pour into a spray bottle or pump, then apply to your clean, dry skin.

Rose Infused Moisturizer

This moisturizer is rich in antioxidants, vitamins, and essential fatty acids, which can help nourish and hydrate the skin.

Ingredients:

- 1/4 cup rose-infused apricot oil
- 1/4 cup jojoba oil
- 1 teaspoon carrot seed oil
- 2 tablespoons mango butter
- 2 tablespoons beeswax
- 1 tablespoon rosehip seed oil
- 10 drops rose essential oil
- 10 drops geranium essential oil
- 5 drops lavender essential oil
- 5 drops frankincense essential oil

Here are some other essential oil blends you might like to try: For **dry skin**: lavender, geranium, and sandalwood. For skin with **acne**: tea tree, lavender, and lemon. For **sensitive skin**: chamomile, lavender, and rose. For **mature skin**: frankincense, rose, and myrrh. For **combination skin**: geranium, lavender, and ylang-ylang.

If you do not have these essential oils feel free to add your favorites or leave them out entirely.

Directions:

1. In a double boiler, melt the mango butter, beeswax, and jojoba oil together until fully melted.
2. Remove from heat and allow the mixture to cool for a few minutes.
3. Stir in the rose-infused apricot oil, rosehip seed oil, and carrot seed oil.
4. Add the essential oils and mix well.
5. Pour the mixture into a clean, sterilized jar or tin.
6. Allow the moisturizer to cool and solidify before using.
7. To use, scoop a small amount of the moisturizer and warm it between your fingertips. Apply to your face or body, massaging gently into the skin.

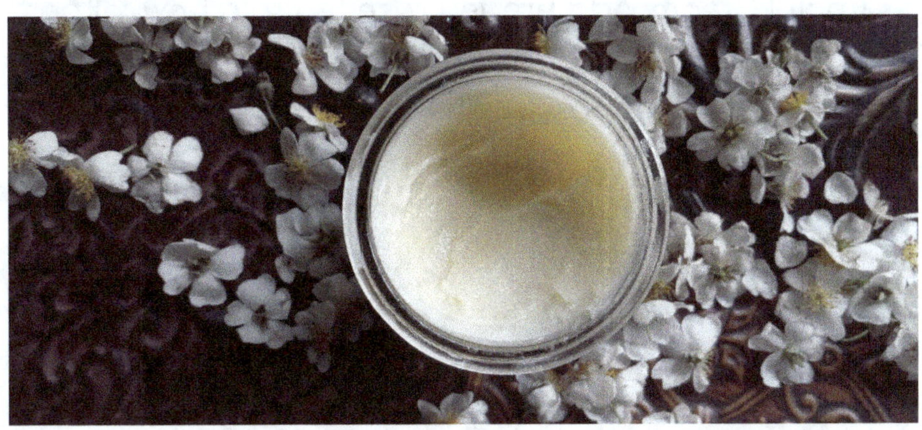

Rose Tea for Self-Care

I love rose tea! I love white rose tea, or black tea or lavender rose mint tea. Basically, I will drink any tea that has roses! Here are a few of my favorites: Numi white rose tea, organic India tulsi cinnamon rose, Organic India tulsi sweet rose, English rose black tea and Bigelow rose and mint tea.

Rose tea can be a soothing and aromatic addition to your self-care routine. Here are some ways you can use rose tea for self-care:

Relaxing Bath: Brew a strong pot of rose tea and add it to your bathwater for a relaxing and fragrant soak. The scent of roses can help calm your mind and promote relaxation.

Facial Steam: Add brewed rose tea to a bowl of hot water and use it for a facial steam. The steam can help open up your pores and hydrate your skin, leaving it feeling refreshed. You can create a facial steam blend. Some other botanicals that mix well with rose are dandelion, mint, wild violet, lavender, chamomile, hibiscus, and green tea.

Hair Rinse: Use cooled rose tea as a final rinse after shampooing your hair. The natural oils in rose petals can help condition your hair and leave it smelling lovely.

Eye Compress: Soak cotton pads in cooled rose tea and place them over your eyes for a soothing eye compress. This can help reduce puffiness and refresh tired eyes.

Scented Spray: Pour brewed and cooled rose tea into a spray bottle and use it as a natural room or linen spray. The delicate scent of roses can help create a calming atmosphere. You can also use it as a body spray, hair conditioner spray, or facial toner.

Drinking Tea: Of course, one of the most common ways to use rose tea is to drink it. Rose tea is often enjoyed for its calming properties and delicate flavor. You can drink it hot or cold, depending on your preference.

Rose Mint Bath tea

This bath tea is not only aromatic but also offers potential benefits for the skin and senses. The combination of ingredients can help soothe the skin, relax the mind, and create a luxurious bathing experience. Adjust the quantities based on your preference and the size of your bathtub.

Ingredients:

- 1/4 cup dried rose petals
- 1/4 cup dried mint leaves
- 2-3 green tea bags or 2 tablespoons loose green tea
- Optional: 1/4 cup Epsom salt or sea salt

Directions:

1. Combine the dried rose petals, mint leaves, and green tea in a bowl.
2. If using, add the Epsom salt or sea salt to the mixture and stir to combine.
3. Spoon the mixture into a muslin bag, teabags, or a clean, old sock, and tie it closed securely.
4. Hang the bag under the faucet as you fill the bathtub with hot water. Allow the bag to steep in the water as the tub fills.
5. Once the tub is filled, remove the bag and discard it.
6. Enjoy your relaxing bath infused with the soothing scents of roses, mint, and green tea.

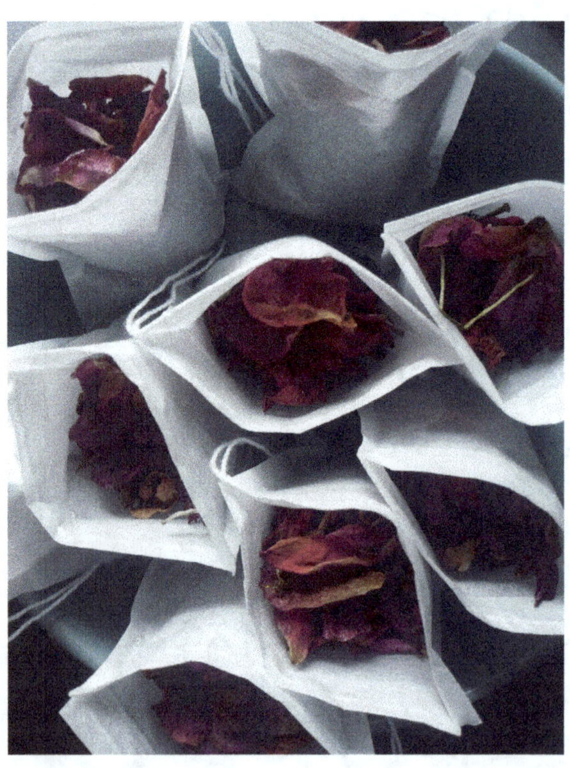

Milk Baths

When was the last time you took a milk bath? A milk bath is a bath that has milk as its main ingredient. Other ingredients typically include honey, essential oils, or herbs. Lactic acid, a component of milk helps exfoliate and promote cell turnover. Milk moisturizes dry skin, soothes sunburn, and is very relaxing.

People have been indulging in milk baths since ancient times as they are luxurious and skin nourishing. Cleopatra was known for loving milk baths as it helped maintain her beauty and keep her skin soft. According to a legend, she bathed in donkey's milk, honey, and almond oil. Greeks and Romans also enjoyed milk baths because they believed that milk could soothe and heal the skin and help with its texture.

Milks

Milk baths can make your skin feel soft and smooth. It will be gently exfoliated. They smell nice and feel luxurious and help us to relax. There are different types of milk of course. Their benefits will differ. You can use cow's milk powder which is readily available in your local grocery store. You can also use goat's milk powder. It has a higher percentage of butter fat so it will feel creamier and more luxurious.

You can also use nut milks if you are a vegan. I like to use coconut milk powder. It has a lovely smell and feels so nice. It is moisturizing and nourishing and can help prevent dryness and wrinkles.

Clays

Clay is the most used ingredient in a detox bath as it is great in drawing toxins out of the body. Bentonite clay is the most used for baths but there are many different ones. There was a study done at Arizona State University in which it was concluded that bentonite clay could kill Staphylococcus, MRSA, E. coli and other pathogens. Clay can also help with digestive issues, skin allergies, sinus problems, headaches, and helps you recover from diarrhea and vomiting.

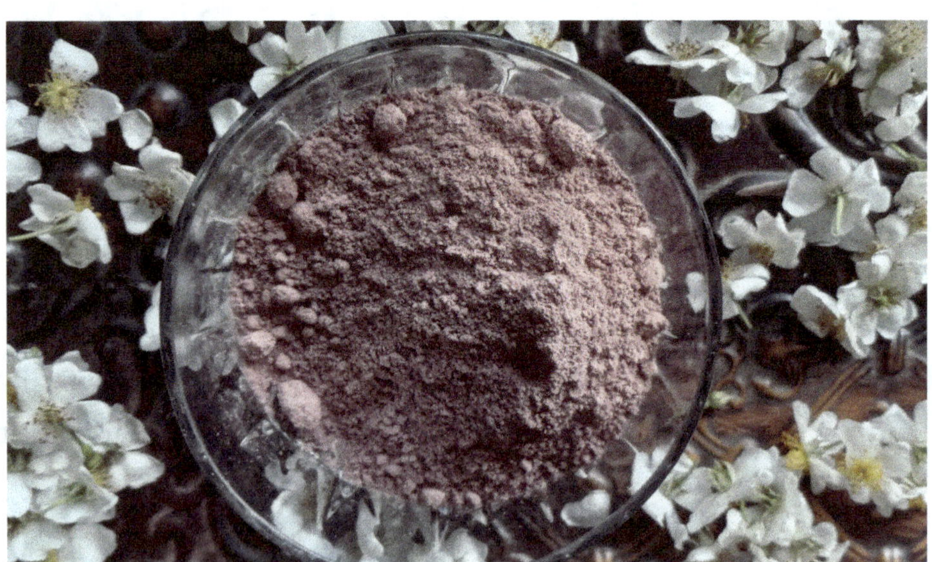

Other Ingredients

Citrus

Slice up any citrus fruit in thick slices and toss in the bath. The vitamin C and citric acid in citrus fruits help circulation and shrink pores.

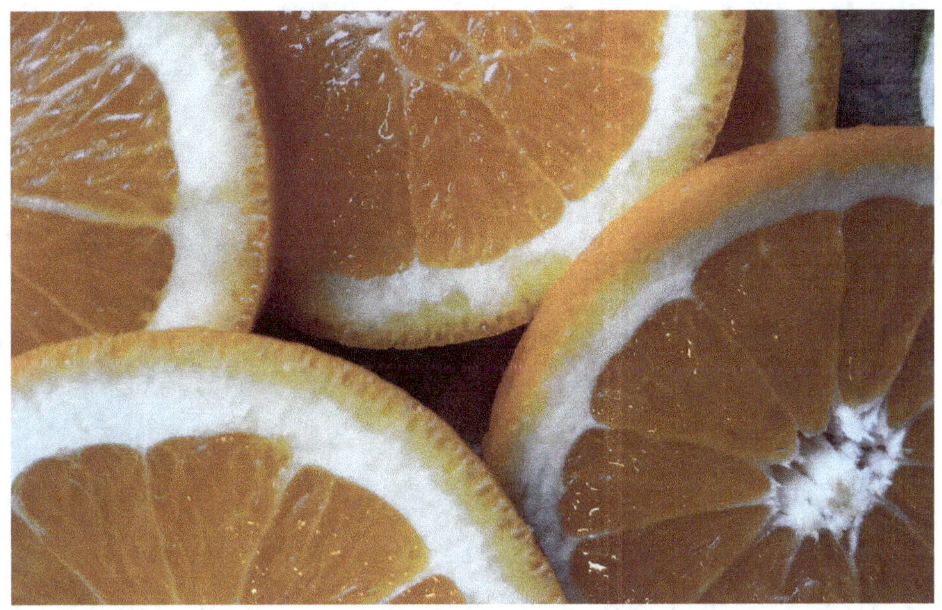

Oatmeal

Soothing, moisturizing and anti-inflammatory. Is great for soothing itchy and sensitive skin.

Vinegar

Helps kill bacterial infections, helps get rid of body odor, is good for hair and skin health and foot issues such as athlete's foot, foot odor, and warts according to Medical News Today.

Aloe Vera

Aloe Vera can be used as a carrier for essential oils. Is great for sunburn, eczema and other skin irritations.

Rice Powder

Helps absorb excess oil, helps shed dead skin cells, is anti-aging, helps treat acne, is antioxidant, anti-inflammatory and anti-microbial.

Baking soda

Baking soda is amazing for cleansing and detoxifying your whole body, boosting your immune system and eliminating any toxin build-up. It helps soothe eczema, works with Epsom salts to help sore muscles and helps to eliminate odor.

Flowers and Herbs

When using flowers and herbs in the bath, you can use them fresh and put them directly in the bath or you can use them dried and either put them directly in the bath or make a tea out of them first and pour it in the bathtub.

To make tea with them, boil them in 8 cups of water, reduce heat and simmer until half the water has evaporated, strain the water and add to your bath.

Rose Bath Milk

This bath milk is nourishing for the skin and provides a luxurious bathing experience. The combination of ingredients helps to soften and moisturize the skin while the soothing scents of roses create a relaxing atmosphere. Adjust the quantities based on your preference and the size of your bathtub.

Ingredients:

- 1/2 cup dried rose petals
- 1/2 cup coconut milk powder
- 1/2 cup oatmeal
- Optional: a few drops of rose essential oil for extra fragrance

Instructions:

1. Grind the dried rose petals and oatmeal in a blender, coffee grinder or food processor until they form a fine powder.
2. In a bowl, mix the ground rose petals and oatmeal with the coconut milk powder.
3. Add a few drops of rose essential oil if desired, for extra fragrance.
4. To use, simply add a few tablespoons of the bath milk to warm running water and swirl to dissolve. Enjoy a soothing and moisturizing bath infused with the scents of roses, coconut, and oatmeal.

Milk Bath

Ingredients:

2 cups milk powder

1 cup oat flour or ¼ cup rice powder

Up to ½ cup honey powder, kaolin clay or cornstarch

2 tbsp dried flowers

¼ cup Salt or baking soda

Essential oils

Directions: Mix dry ingredients, add essential oils and stir well. Store in an airtight jar.

Use 2 to 4 tbsp per bath.

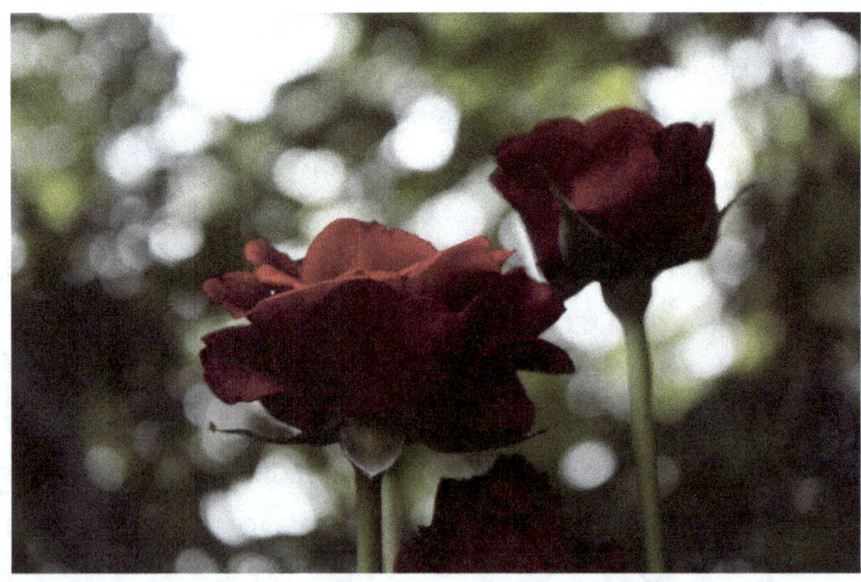

Rose Body Scrub

Arrowroot Powder

Absorbs Excess Moisture:

Arrowroot powder is effective at absorbing excess moisture on the skin like sebum. This can be especially beneficial for people who have oily or combination skin.

Gentle Exfoliation:

Arrowroot powder can gently exfoliate the skin when used in facial masks or scrubs. It helps with the removal of dead skin cells, which leaves the skin glowing and feeling smoother.

Soothing and Healing:

Arrowroot powder is very soothing to the skin, especially when it is irritated or inflamed. It may be helpful in calming redness and helping in the healing of minor skin irritations.

Suitable for Sensitive Skin:

Arrowroot powder is generally considered gentle and can be used by people with sensitive skin. It is used a lot in baby products instead of talcum powder.

Citric Acid

Mild Exfoliator

Using citric acid in your skincare can help improve its texture and appearance as it is a mild exfoliator.

May not be Good for Sensitive Skin

Do not use citric acid if you have sensitive skin as it can be harsh for some skin. It is also possible to be allergic to citric acid.

Epsom Salt

Epsom Salt does not have sodium chloride in it, so it is not a real salt. However, it does have magnesium, sulfur and oxygen and looks like salt. It is good for getting rid of toxins, exfoliating, and relieving stress and muscle pain.

Sea Salt

Sea salt is naturally occurring and one of the most used salts for bath salts. It comes from the evaporation of seawater and its grains are larger than those of table salt. It can be refined or unrefined. Refined sea salt has been washed so unrefined is generally recommended. Sea Salt baths help relieve stress, ease achy muscles, and treat irritated skin.

Rose Body Scrub

Ingredients:

- 1/2 cup dried rose petals
- 1/4 cup fresh mint leaves, chopped
- 1 cup granulated sugar
- 1/2 cup coconut oil, melted
- 1 teaspoon vanilla extract

Instructions:

1. Grind the dried rose petals and fresh mint leaves in a blender or food processor until they are finely chopped.
2. In a bowl, combine the chopped rose petals and mint leaves with the granulated sugar.
3. Add the melted coconut oil and vanilla extract to the sugar mixture and stir until well combined.
4. Transfer the body scrub to a clean, airtight container for storage.

To use, simply take a small amount of the scrub and massage it onto damp skin in a gentle, circular motion. Rinse off with warm water. The sugar will exfoliate the skin, while the coconut oil will moisturize. The scent of roses, mint, and vanilla will create a luxurious and invigorating experience. Adjust the quantities based on your preference and the size of the container you use for storage.

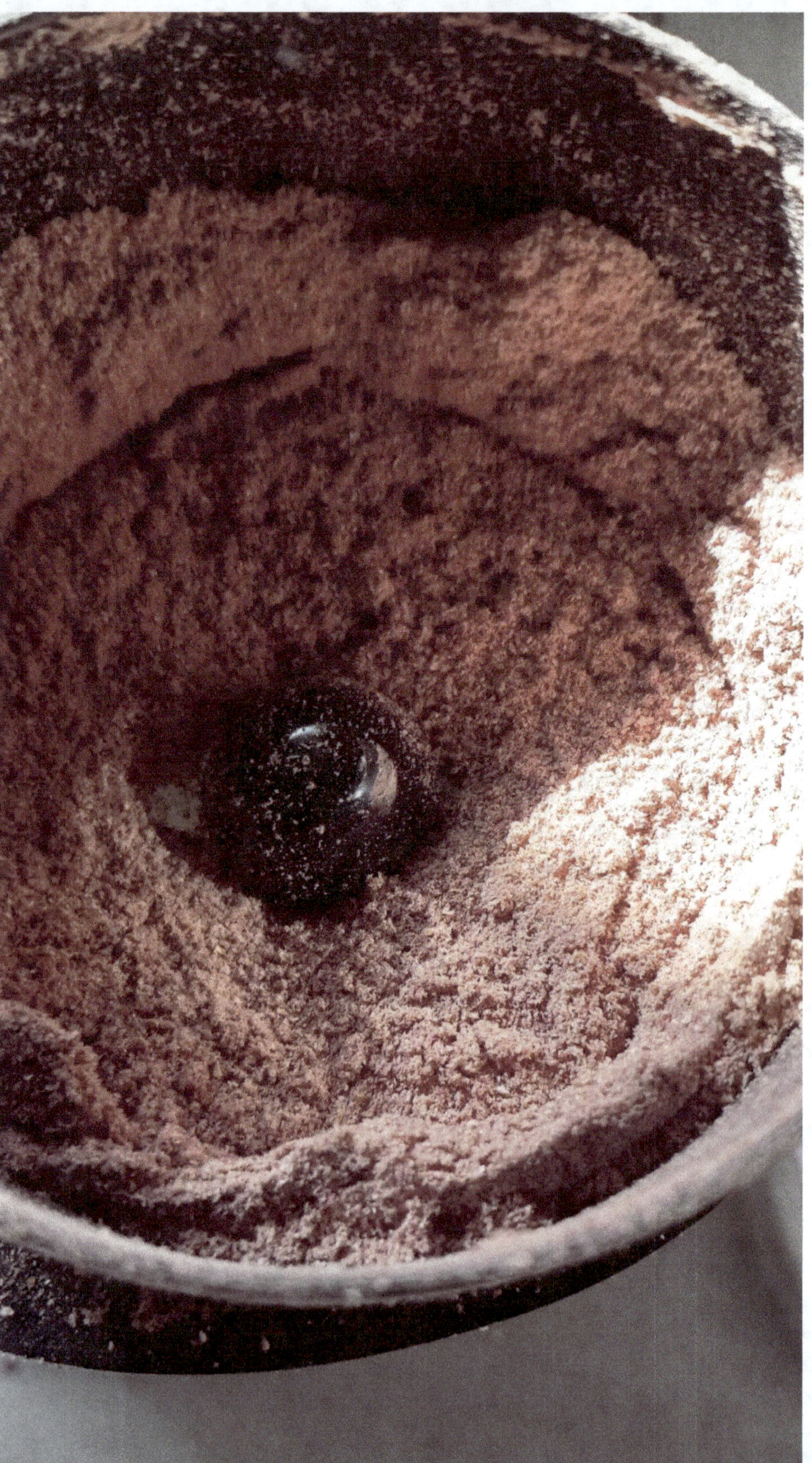

Relaxing Rose Body Scrub:

Ingredients:

- 1 cup Epsom salt
- 1/2 cup Himalayan Sea salt
- 1/4 cup sea salt
- 1/4 cup dried and powdered roses (I use a coffee grinder)
- 2 tablespoons citric acid
- 2 tablespoons arrowroot powder
- 1/2 cup grapeseed oil (or your favorite oil)
- 15 drops essential oil

Directions:

1. **Mix the Salts Together:** In a mixing bowl, combine the rose powder, Epsom salt, Himalayan Sea salt, and sea salt. Stir the salts together to ensure an even distribution.
2. **Add Citric Acid and Arrowroot Powder:** Add the citric acid and arrowroot powder to the salt mixture. These ingredients can add a gentle exfoliating and softening effect to the scrub.
3. **Stir in The Grapeseed Oil:** Pour the grapeseed oil over the salt mixture. Mix well to create a wet, granulated texture. Adjust the amount of grapeseed oil based on your desired consistency.

4. **Add Essential Oils:** Add 15 drops of essential oil to the mixture.

5. **Stir Thoroughly:** Stir the ingredients thoroughly to ensure that the essential oils are evenly distributed throughout the scrub.

6. **Check Consistency:** Check the consistency of the scrub. If it's too dry, add a bit more grapeseed oil; if it's too wet, add a little more salt.

7. **Transfer to a Jar:** Transfer the body scrub into a clean, airtight jar or container for storage. Make sure to seal the container tightly after each use to keep the scrub fresh.

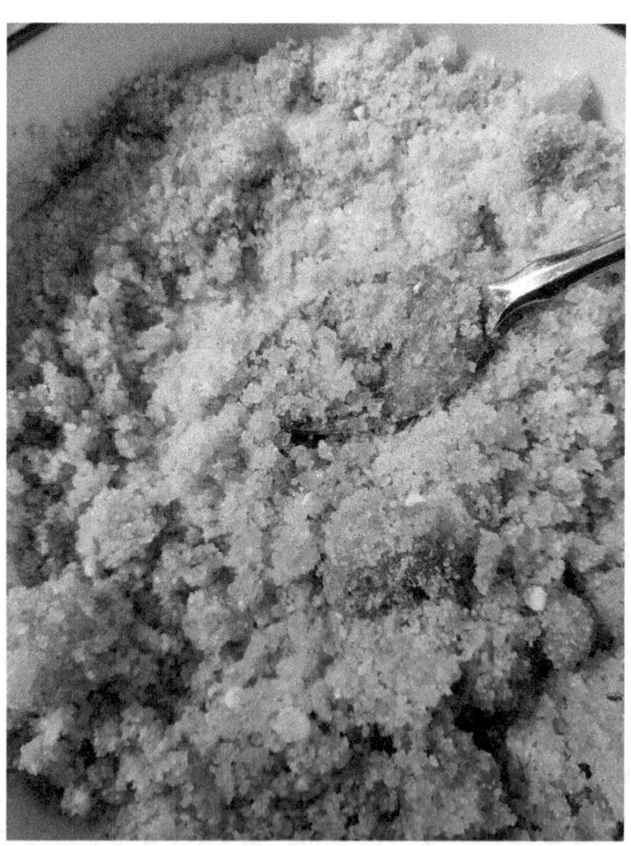

Moisturizing Lip Balm

Lip balm is a thing I get excited about. It's my best seller. I first started making it because the stuff I was using just wasn't moisturizing.

"I LOVE these lip balms! I have tried several throughout the years and these lip balms are the only ones that I have found that truly moisturize!" - Jessica C.

So, if you would like to make your own moisturizing lip balm, then this chapter is for you.

Beeswax

What is Beeswax? It is wax made from bees used to store the colonies' honey.

Uses: It is in many products including makeup, baby products, sunscreen, lip balm, moisturizers etc.

Benefits: Beeswax will create a protective layer on the skin. It is a humectant and a moisturizing, hydrating, soothing, natural exfoliator.

Risks: Before using beeswax, you may want to test for allergies.

For beeswax, you want to use about 4 times as much oil as wax. If you want to use essential oils, remember to use 1% essential oils and add them in at the end. Have fun experimenting with ingredients. You can try different oils, butters, colorants, etc.

Soy Wax

What is soy wax? Soy wax is a natural and renewable wax derived from soybean oil.

Uses: Soy wax can be used in a variety of cosmetics and hair care products, such as lip balms, lotions, lipsticks, body butters, creams, lotion bars, and hair pomades and also candles.

Benefits: Soy wax is made from soybeans, which are a renewable resource. It is a good vegan wax for using in lip balms because of its natural emollient and moisturizing properties.

Risks: While soy allergies are relatively uncommon, they can happen. Some people may have sensitive skin that reacts to certain ingredients, including soy-based products. You might want to perform a patch test before applying soy wax or products containing soy wax to a larger area of the skin. Most commercially available soy wax is made from genetically modified soybeans. If you prefer non-GMO products, you may want to look for soy wax specifically labeled as non-GMO or choose alternative waxes.

Oils for Lips

When you are choosing oils for your lips, it's important to choose oils that are nourishing, hydrating, and suitable for the delicate skin on the lips. Here are some oils commonly used in lip care products:

Coconut Oil:

Coconut oil is known for its moisturizing properties and helps prevent moisture loss and keeps lips soft. It also has antimicrobial properties.

Jojoba Oil:

Jojoba oil closely resembles sebum, the natural oils in our skin, making it easily absorbed. It helps to hydrate and soothe dry lips.

Sweet Almond Oil:

Rich in vitamin E, sweet almond oil is an emollient that helps soften and nourish the skin. It's gentle and suitable for sensitive skin.

Olive Oil:

Olive oil is high in antioxidants and contains healthy fats. It helps moisturize and protect the lips from dryness.

Avocado Oil:

Avocado oil is rich in fatty acids and vitamin E, providing deep hydration and promoting softness. It's particularly beneficial for extremely dry or chapped lips.

Argan Oil:

Argan oil is rich in antioxidants and essential fatty acids, making it a good choice for moisturizing and protecting the lips.

Rosehip Seed Oil:

Rosehip seed oil is high in vitamin C and promotes skin regeneration. It can help repair and rejuvenate chapped lips.

Grapeseed Oil:

Grapeseed oil is lightweight and absorbs quickly, making it a good option for a non-greasy feel. It contains antioxidants and vitamins.

Butters

Cocoa Butter

Cocoa butter is an excellent facial moisturizer and prevents dryness and peeling. It heals chapped lips. It is an emollient. This means it protects lips by adding a protective moisturizing layer to them. Cocoa butter helps skin elasticity, skin tone, and collagen retention and production. It is gentle and good at soothing burns, rashes, infections, and things like eczema or dermatitis. It is also beneficial to use cocoa butter as a pre-shave lotion to prevent nicks from occurring and to have softer skin.

Mango Butter

Mango butter contains natural antioxidants, vitamins A and E, and essential fatty acids. Mango butter moisturizes dry skin, itchy skin, skin rashes and peeling. It moisturizes and smooths rough skin, small skin wounds and skin cracks. It works on fine lines and wrinkles, blemishes, and stretch marks. Use it in a shaving cream for a smooth shave. It treats sunburn, insect bites, poison ivy, poison oak, eczema and dermatitis.

Shea Butter

Shea butter has a high concentration of vitamin, antioxidants and fatty acids including linoleic, oleic, stearic, and palmitic acids. It is antifungal and antibacterial, so it helps fight skin infections and the bacteria on the skin. It is anti- inflammatory which helps for things like wind-blown skin and eczema. It is good for all skin types. Antioxidants help shea butter to protect your skin from free radicals which lead to premature aging. It may help acne, fine lines and wrinkles. It may help prevent hair breakage and dandruff. Shea butter may also help sunburn, eczema, dermatitis, psoriasis, wounds, and insect bites.

Simple Moisturizing Lip Balm

Ingredients:

4 tsp Coconut oil

4 tsp rose infused almond Oil

2 tsp beeswax

Shea Butter Lip Balm

Ingredients:

4 tsp Shea butter

4 tsp rose infused coconut oil

2 tsp beeswax

4 drops vitamin E

Directions:

1. In a double boiler, melt the coconut oil, beeswax pellets, and shea butter together until fully liquid.
2. Remove from heat and let it cool slightly.
3. Add your chosen essential oil blend and stir well.
4. Pour the mixture into lip balm containers (using plastic pipettes) or small jars.
5. Allow the lip balm to cool and solidify before using.

Rose Tinted Lip Balm

Ingredients:

- 2 tablespoons rose-infused olive oil
- 1 tablespoon coconut oil
- 1 tablespoon cocoa butter
- 1 tablespoon beeswax
- 1/2 teaspoon rosehip seed powder (optional, for a hint of color)

Directions:

1. In a double boiler, melt the rose-infused olive oil, coconut oil, cocoa butter, and beeswax together until fully melted.
2. Stir in the rosehip seed powder, if using, and mix well.
3. Pour the mixture into lip balm tubes or tins.
4. Allow the lip balm to cool and solidify before using.
5. To use, apply the lip balm to your lips as needed for hydration and protection.

Make Your Own Rose Infused Oil Roller Ball

A roller ball with oil can be used for many different purposes. I like to use them as a cuticle oil, eye oil, lip oil, face oil, perfume or body oil. You can also make them for uses such as headache, cough, aromatherapy or many other things.

What you will need:

-A roller ball

-Your choice of oil(s)

-Dried flowers or herbs

-Essential Oils

Here are some essential oil blend suggestions: **Floral:** lavender, ylang-ylang, and geranium. **Citrus:** sweet orange, bergamot, and grapefruit. **Woodsy:** cedarwood, sandalwood, and frankincense. **Romantic:** rose, jasmine, and sandalwood. **Fresh and clean:** lemon, lavender, and peppermint. **Spicy:** clove, cinnamon, and orange. **Calm:** patchouli, lavender, and frankincense. **Serene:** Vanilla, lavender, and chamomile.

Directions:

-Add flowers or herbs to the bottle.

-Drop in essential oils. If you are using it on your face (including lips), you'll want to use 1% essential oils which is 2 drops. If you wish to make a blend of several essential oils, you can combine them in a separate container then use a dropper to put them in your rollerball. If you are using it for your body, use 2% essential oils which would be 4 drops. If you are using it for a headache, you can use 5% which is 5 drops.

-Pour in oils.

-Put the roller ball on and use your oil.

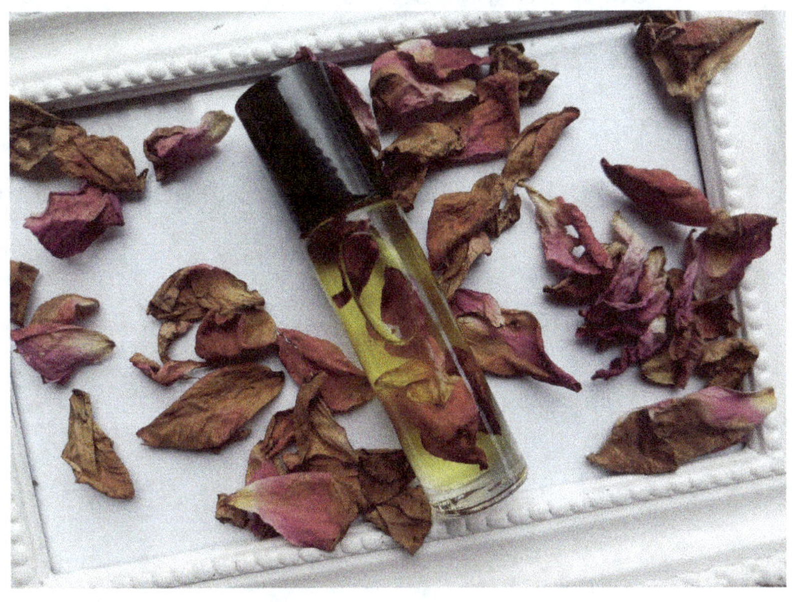

Colorful Bath Bomb Recipe

Do you love bath bombs but hate that the really good ones are so expensive? Try this recipe below to make your own personalized bath bombs. Try different colors and fragrances and have fun!

Rose Bath Bomb

Ingredients:

- 1 cup baking soda
- 1/2 cup citric acid
- 1/2 cup Epsom salts
- 1/2 cup cornstarch
- 2 tablespoons rose powder
- 2 tablespoons coconut oil, melted
- 1 teaspoon water
- 10-20 drops of rose essential oil (optional, for fragrance)
- Bath bomb molds

Directions:

1. In a large bowl, mix together the baking soda, citric acid, Epsom salts, cornstarch, and rose powder.
2. In a separate small bowl, mix together the melted coconut oil, water, and rose essential oil (if using).
3. VERY Slowly add the liquid mixture to the dry ingredients, stirring constantly to avoid fizzing.
4. The mixture should hold together when squeezed without crumbling. If it's too dry, add a little more water, a few drops at a time.
5. Firmly pack the mixture into bath bomb molds and let them dry for at least 24 hours.
6. Carefully remove the bath bombs from the molds and store them in an airtight container until ready to use.

To make them more fun:

Use gel food coloring or bath bomb colorants for bright colors.

Add dried flowers or herbs to the molds before putting in the bath bomb mixture, to make the bath bombs even prettier and more beneficial.

Experiment with different essential oil blends with different scents and benefits.

Here are some essential oil blends you might want to try:

1) Relaxing: Lavender and chamomile.
2) Energizing: Orange, lemon and grapefruit.
3) Floral: Geranium, ylang-ylang, and rose.
4) Refreshing: Peppermint, eucalyptus, and tea tree.
5) Vanilla Citrus: Vanilla, sweet orange, and bergamot.
6) Uplifting: Rose, geranium, and bergamot.
7) Sensual: Jasmine, ylang-ylang, and sandalwood.

Crafting Your Own Luxurious Body Powder

Body Powder

Body powder is something that not many people use anymore but can be very helpful. It is a multi-purpose product. I will give you some ideas and a recipe and tell you about a few of the ingredients. You can use it right after the bath as a deodorant, to prevent chafing, and give your skin a nice scent. You can use them on the baby's bottom (and your own). You can also make a powder to use as a dry shampoo.

There are many different ingredients to pick and choose from. For the base of the powder, you can use cornstarch, arrowroot powder, or baking soda. Then you add clay, oat flour, or rice flour. You can use dried herbs or flowers such as spearmint or roses. I also like to use zinc oxide as it is anti-aging and a great deodorant.

Body Powder Bases

Arrowroot Powder

Arrowroot powder is beneficial for all skin types and is softening and smoothing. It is gentle on sensitive skin and is anti-inflammatory.

Arrowroot powder contains helpful ingredients such as zinc, iron, potassium, and vitamin B6. It can help skin with rashes, acne or sores. It is a good skin conditioner and oil reducer. Arrowroot powder can help improve your skin's texture and help you get the glowing skin you want.

Baking Soda

Baking soda is antiseptic and antibacterial therefore it may help get rid of the bacteria that causes acne; however, not the acne on your face. It is a good treatment for the back or shoulders. It is a natural deodorant, balances PH, and soothes irritation. Baking soda has natural exfoliating properties that can help remove dead skin cells and unclog pores, leaving the skin smoother and brighter. If you have sensitive skin, do a patch test first as it can be harsh on the skin.

Cornstarch

Cornstarch is a natural and safe ingredient that has great absorbent properties and can help keep the skin dry and comfortable. It is gentle on the skin and can soothe irritation. It helps reduce friction by absorbing moisture. It has a smooth texture which can help give body powder that silky smooth feeling.

kaolin Clay

Clay has many benefits for skin care. Clays are bactericidal, antiseptic and balancing.

They help cell turnover, healing, softening, help acne, and managing excess oil. There are different types of kaolin clay that work better with different types of skin including white, red, yellow and pink. If you have sensitive or dry skin, use white clay. For oily skin and acne, use red clay as it is the most absorbing. Yellow clay is absorbing and exfoliating but is still fine for sensitive skin. Pink is a mix of white and red and is good for delicate skin.

Body Powder Botanical Extras

Chamomile

Chamomile is gentle and soothing and a great ingredient for sensitive skin. It can help calm inflamed and irritated skin. It is also great for dry and itchy skin.

Calendula

Calendula is another plant that is great for soothing and healing the skin as it has anti-inflammatory and antibacterial properties.

Lavender

Everyone knows lavender is soothing and calming and smells lovely. Use it if you want a relaxing body powder after your bath.

Rose

With its smell and color, roses make a lovely body powder for after your bath. Rose can help to soften and moisturize the skin.

Rosemary

Rosemary has high antioxidant and antimicrobial activity. It's a great addition to your body powder, deodorant, or dry shampoo. It can benefit your hair and scalp in many ways. It stimulates hair growth, helps prevent dandruff, strengthens hair, adds shine, and soothes irritation.

Spearmint

Spearmint is a good choice for deodorant as it has antibacterial and antimicrobial properties. It is soothing and refreshing. It can help skin problems such as insect bites or burns.

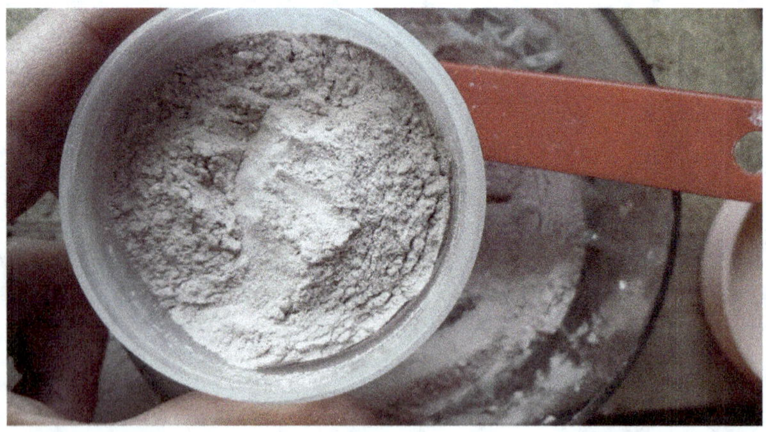

10 Ways You Can Use Body Powder

Depending on what you want to use the powder for, you might want to add different ingredients. For instance, for a deodorant you might want to add mint and zinc oxide. For a dry shampoo, you might want to add rosemary or mint.

1. As a Deodorant
2. After your shower or bath
3. Before exercise on areas prone to chafing
4. As a dry shampoo
5. On feet and shoes
6. For baby care
7. As a setting powder
8. In shoes and boots
9. As a scented sachet
10. After waxing or shaving

Rose Body Powder Recipe

1 cup arrowroot powder

½ to ¾ cup kaolin clay

2 tbsp non-nano zinc oxide powder

2 or 3 tbsp rose powder

Mix all ingredients and blend together. Pour them into your favorite container such as powder puff containers, shakers, squeeze bottles, talcum powder containers, or reuse one of your old containers.

Natural Rose Clay for Skin

Clay is a rock or soil material made of aluminum and iron silicates, magnesium, copper, sodium, potassium, and manganese. Use clay in masks and body wraps, or to treat dermatitis caused by poison ivy and poison oak and diaper rash. The benefits of clay include that it is bactericidal, antiseptic, and balancing, and helps cell turnover. It is also healing and softening, prevents acne, and manages excess oil. Be careful as clays may stain fabric. There are many different types of clay but my favorite is rose clay.

Rose kaolin clay can remove toxins from the skin as it exfoliates and polishes the skin. It will gently cleanse the skin, which makes it great for all skin types, even sensitive skin. It is a mild clay that can come from Brazil, Bulgaria, France, the United Kingdom, Iran, Germany, India, Australia, and other countries. It is fine and light and absorbs excess oil.

To help treat acne, make a paste with clay, aloe gel, and tea tree essential oil. Kaolin clay can help tone and tighten the skin.

It is also helpful for the scalp. To make a treatment for your scalp, make a paste out of clay, apple cider vinegar, and lavender Leave it on for 2 minutes and then rinse it off.

Rose Facial Cleansing Powder

ingredients:

½ cup Rice Powder

½ cup Coconut Milk Powder

2 tbsp Rose Clay

1 or 2 tbsp Rose Powder

1 or 2 tbsp Wild Violet Powder

Directions: Mix ingredients and store in a glass jar. Change the amounts of the recipe depending on your skin type. I made this for my skin which is normal to dry. If you have oily skin, you might want to use more clay and less coconut milk powder.

To use: Put about a tablespoon in your hand or a bowl. Add water to make a paste. Apply to your face. Wash off with warm water.

Rose Face Mask

Ingredients:

1 tbsp Colloidal Oatmeal

1 tbsp Rose Clay

2 tbsp Coconut Milk

2 tsp Rose Powder

Directions: Mix ingredients in a bowl. Apply to skin. Let sit for 10 to 15 minutes before washing off.

Rose Lavender Bath Salts

Ingredients:

¼ cup Epsom salts

¼ cup pink Himalayan salt

2 tablespoons coconut milk powder or colloidal oatmeal

1 teaspoon rose kaolin clay

Dried lavender and rose petals

1 tsp carrier oil

Rose and lavender (or your favorite) essential oils

Directions: Mix ingredients together in a bowl. Mix essential oils in carrier oil. Pour them into a glass jar with a lid.

If you enjoyed this book, please consider writing a review on Amazon or Goodreads.

Other books by Carrie Scharf

Carries Herbal Infused Skincare Cookbook: A Beginner's Guide to Creating Your Own Personalized Skincare

Carrie's Herbal Infused Skincare Cookbook: How to Use Herbs and Flowers for Glowing Skin

The Cozy Bath

Skincare for Relaxation

Radiance and Ritual: Skincare and Self-Care for the Winter Season

You can find them here:
amazon.com/author/carriescharf

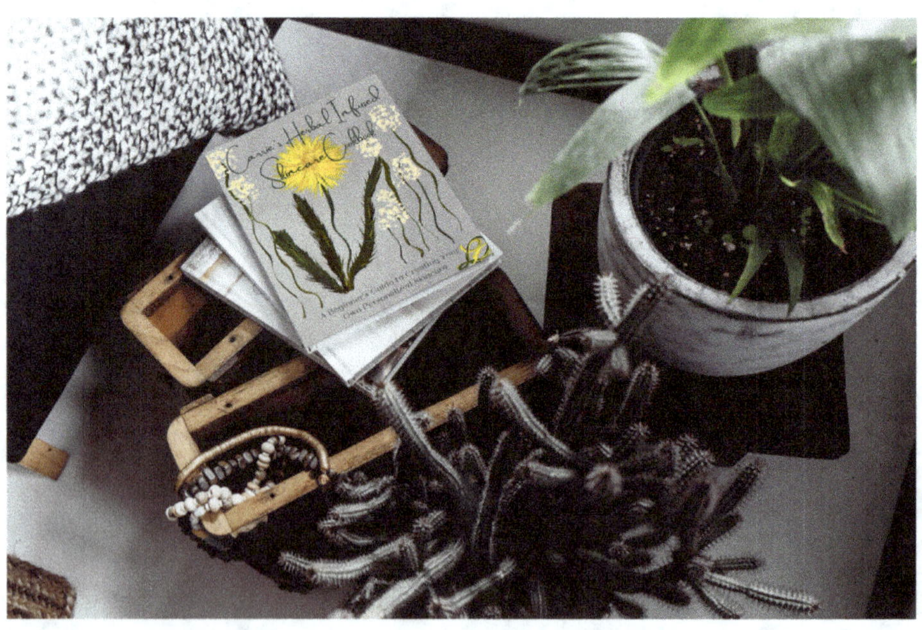